SAFE AND SOUND

A Healthy Body

Angela Royston

Heinemann Library
Des Plaines, Illinois

© 2000 Reed Educational & Professional Publishing
Published by Heinemann Library,
an imprint of Reed Educational & Professional Publishing,
1350 East Touhy Avenue, Suite 240 West
Des Plaines, IL 60018

Customer Service 1-888-454-2279

Text designed by Celia Floyd
Illustrations by Allen Wittert, Pennant Illustration
Printed and bound in Hong Kong, China

04 03 02 01 00
10 9 8 7 6 5 4 3 2 1

Library of Congress Cataloging-in-Publication Data
Royston, Angela.
    A Healthy Body / Royston, Angela.
        p. cm. – (Safe and sound)
    Includes bibliographical references and index.
    Summary: Explains the importance of exercise in maintaining good health and the roles of muscles, joints, heart, and lungs in this process.
    ISBN 1-57572-983-0
    1. Exercise—Physiological aspects Juvenile literature.
2. Physical fitness Juvenile literature. 3. Musculoskeletal system Juvenile literature. [1. Exercise. 2. Physical fitness.]
    I. Title. II. Series: Royston, Angela. Safe and sound.
    QP301.R695 1999
    613.7'1—dc21   99-14554
                                                     CIP

Acknowledgments
The Publishers would like to thank the following for permission to reproduce photographs: Allsport USA/S. Bruty, p. 22; Bubbles/L. Thurston, p. 4; I. West, pp. 10, 11, 13; J. Woodcock, p. 19; J. Allan Cash Ltd., pp. 5, 21; Trevor Clifford, pp. 8, 9, 12, 14, 15, 16, 17, 20, 29; Robert Harding Picture Library, p. 26; Collections/L. Taylor, p. 25; Carol Palmer, p. 23; Tony Stone Images/B. Ayres p. 28.

Cover photo: Trevor Clifford

Every effort has been made to contact copyright holders of any material reproduced in this book. Any omissions will be rectified in subsequent printings if notice is given to the Publisher.

The Publishers would like to thank Julie Johnson, PSHE consultant and trainer, for her comments in the preparation of this book.

Some words in this book are in bold, **like this.** You can find out what they mean by looking in the glossary.

Contents

Healthy Exercise

This girl is chasing her sister. The boys are playing in the sea. They are having fun and **exercising** their bodies.

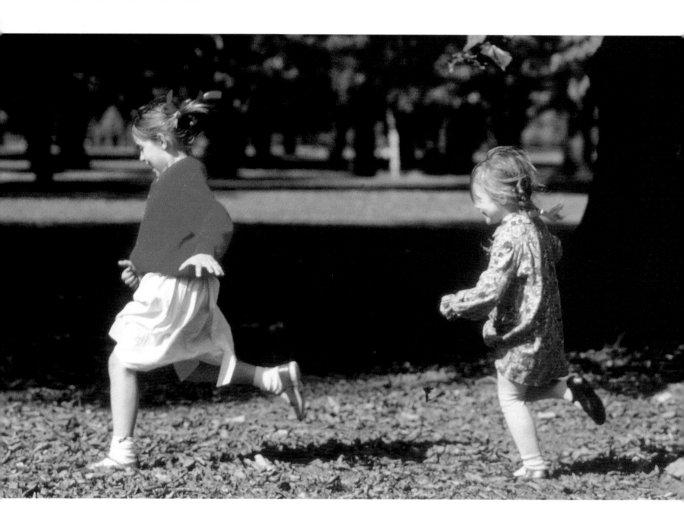

Exercise makes you fit. It keeps your **muscles** strong. It helps your **heart** and **lungs** work well. It keeps your body healthy.

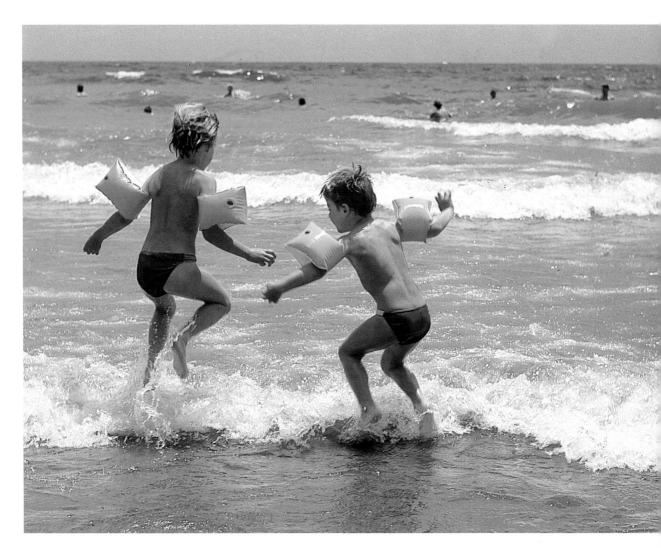

Exercise Pyramid

The **exercise pyramid** shows the **activities** you can do to stay strong and fit. You should spend lots of time doing the kinds of things shown at the bottom of the pyramid. These are called lifestyle activities, because they are the kinds of things you do in your everyday life.

You should spend some time doing the things in the middle of the pyramid. Playing sports and doing **aerobic** activities help keep your **heart** and **lungs** healthy. You also need to do things that will keep you **flexible** and strong.

You need some quiet time, but not too much. Watching television is at the top of the pyramid. It is restful, but it will not make you fit.

6

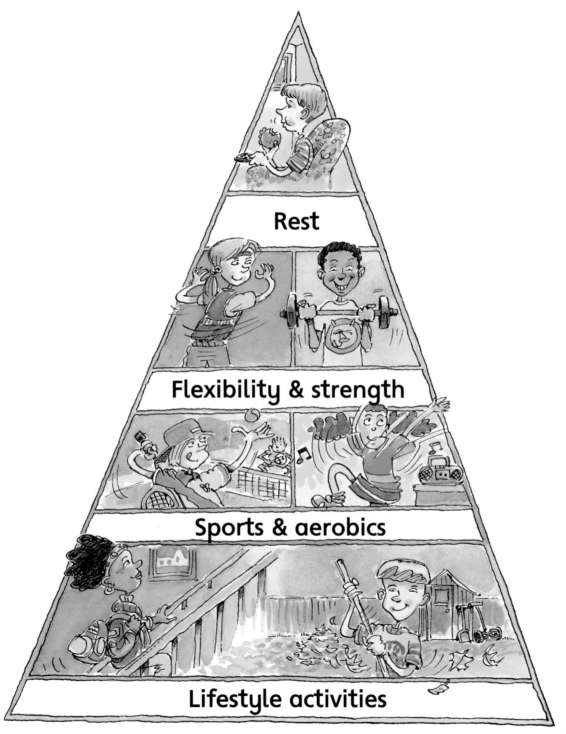

Rest

Flexibility & strength

Sports & aerobics

Lifestyle activities

What Do Muscles Do?

Feel your arm. Can you feel the soft **muscle** and **bone** under your skin? The muscles are connected to the bones. They make the bones move.

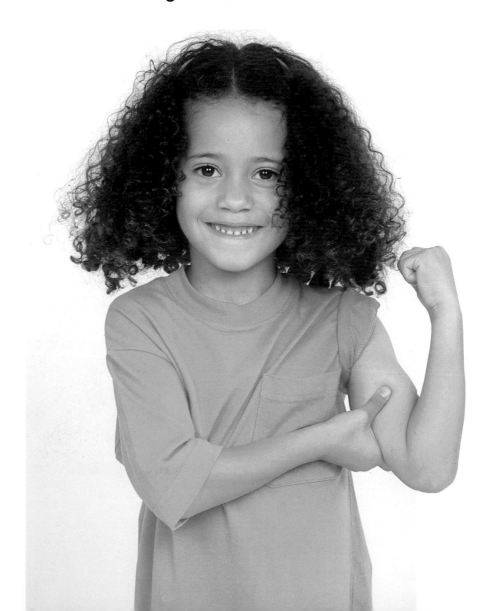

Stretch one of your legs and point your toes.

Can you feel the muscle on the back of your leg?

Stretching helps your muscles get ready for **exercise**.

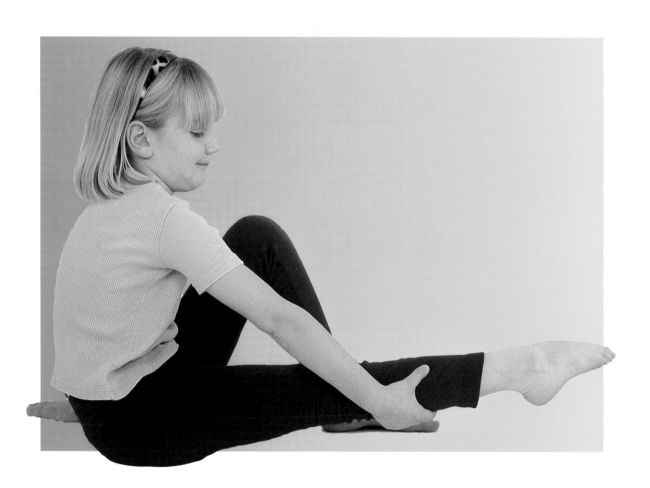

Muscle Power

The more you use your **muscles,** the bigger and stronger they get. Running and kicking a ball makes the muscles in your legs stronger.

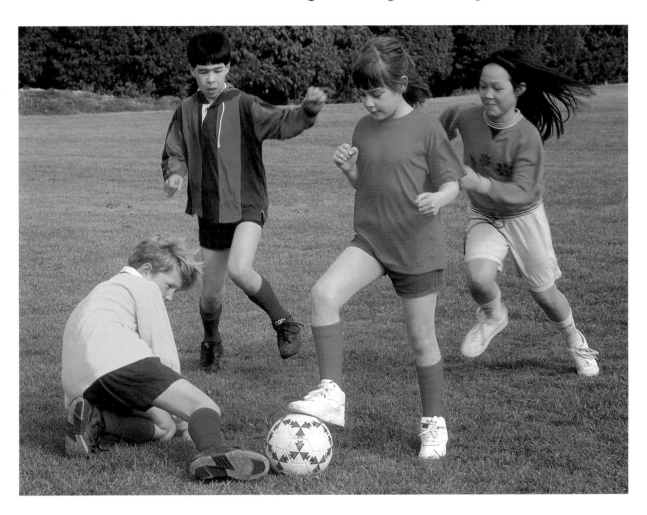

Swimming uses muscles all over your body. You move your legs, arms, back, and head as you swim through the water.

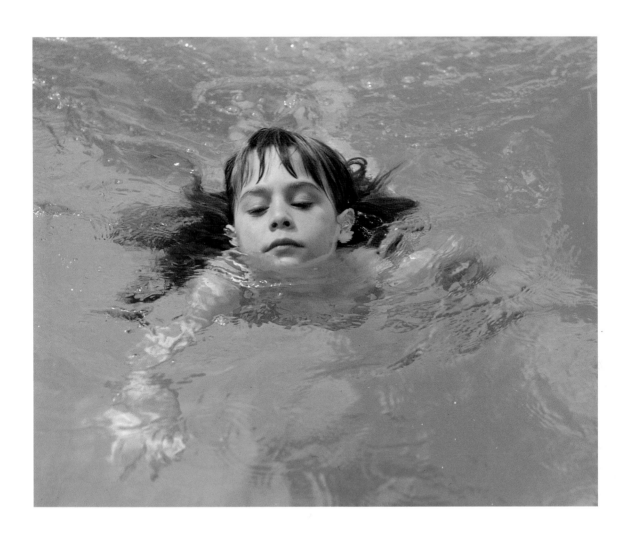

Joints

Bones cannot bend. You can only bend your body at a **joint**. A joint is a place where two bones meet. Here are some of the joints in your body.

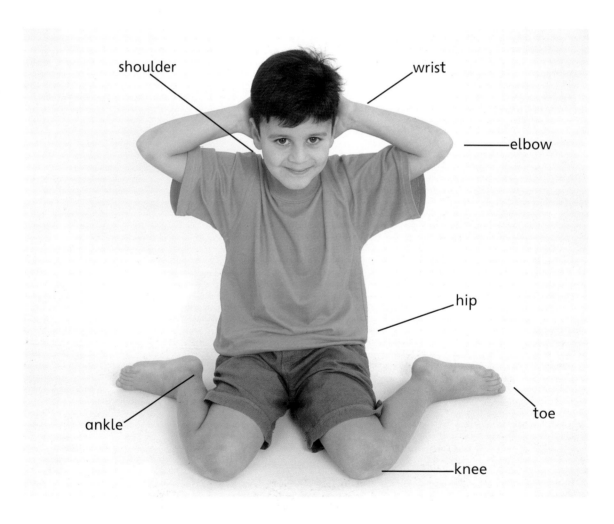

Some joints move in all directions. Some move backward and forward. Climbing on a jungle gym uses joints all over your body.

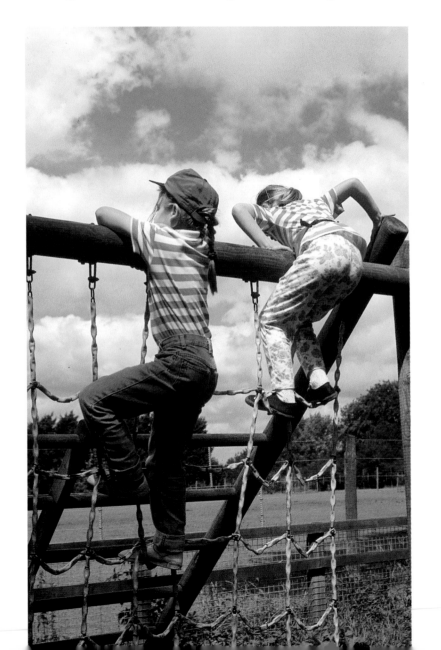

Bending and Stretching

Some people can move their **muscles** and **joints** more than others. You need to be very **flexible** to sit like this.

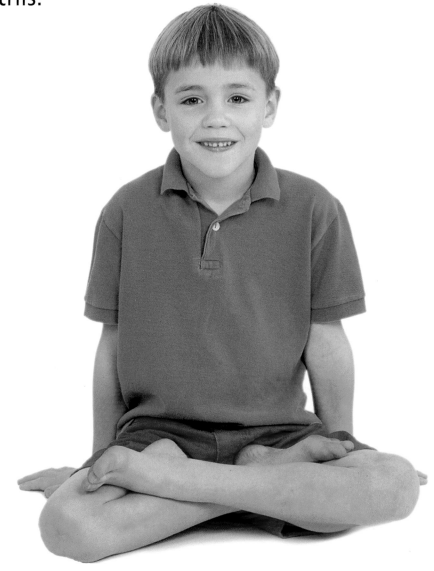

Gymnastics can help you become stronger and more flexible. With practice, you may be able to bend and stretch your whole body!

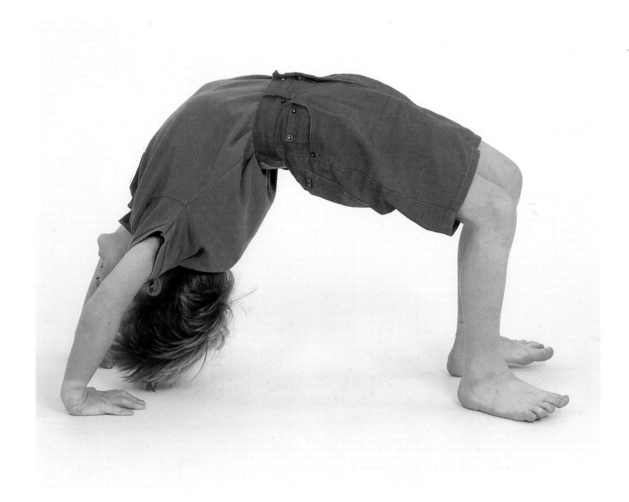

Standing and Lifting

Even when you are standing still, your **joints** and **muscles** are still hard at work. It is better for your muscles when you stand with your back straight.

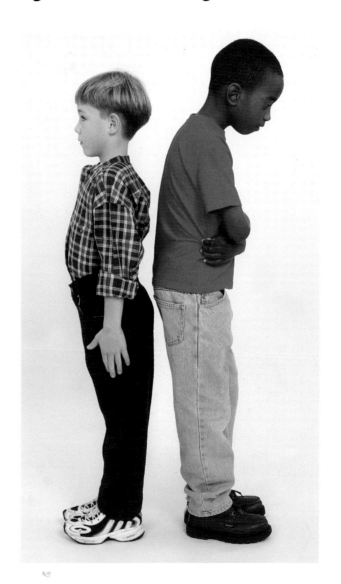

Lifting heavy things can hurt the joints in your back. Always bend your knees and keep your back straight when you lift something heavy.

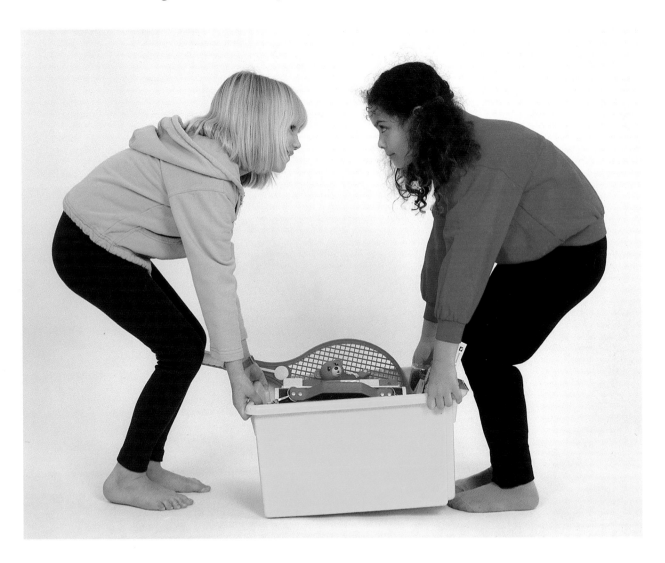

Puffing and Panting

Your body needs **oxygen,** which you breathe into your **lungs**. Your lungs fill with air, just like this balloon.

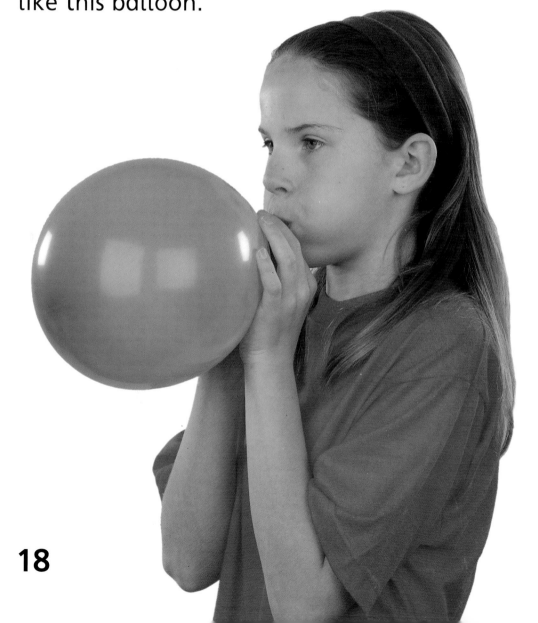

When you run, you use up a lot of oxygen. You may puff and pant as your lungs try to get more oxygen.

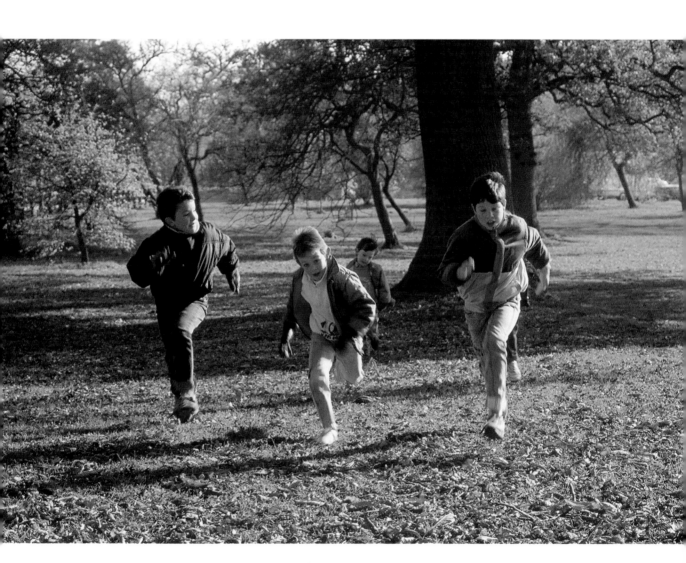

Exercising Your Heart

Your **heart** is a **muscle,** too. Can you feel it beating in your chest? Your heart pumps **blood** around your body. Blood carries food and **oxygen**.

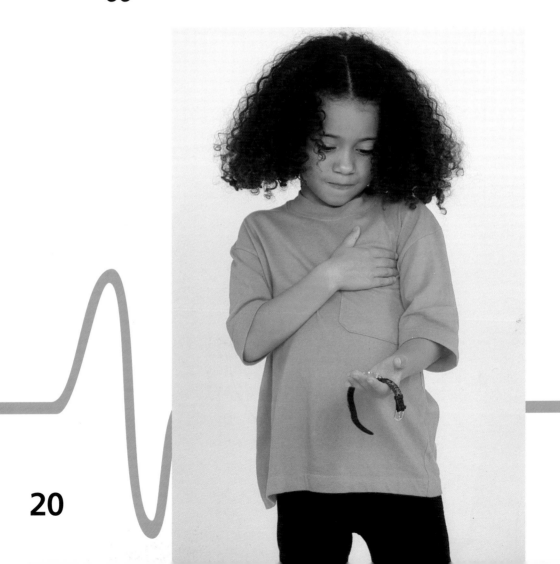

When your muscles work hard, your heart beats faster to give them more oxygen. **Exercise** makes your heart and **lungs** work better. It also makes you hot and thirsty!

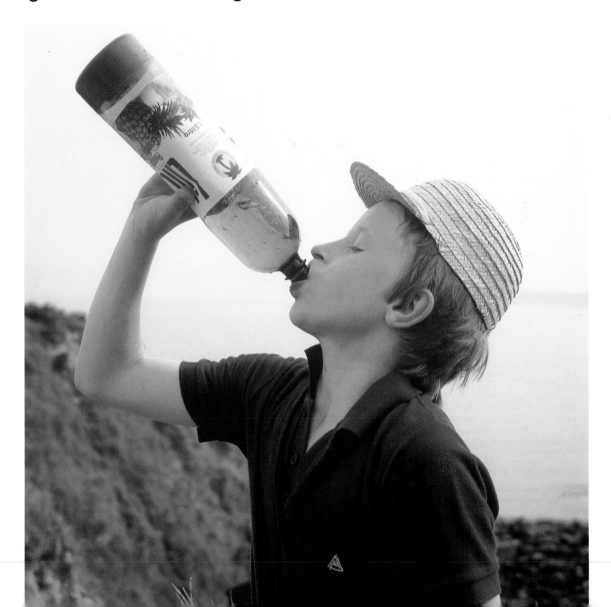

Balancing Act

It is hard to balance when you first begin to skate. It takes lots of practice until your **muscles** get used to working together.

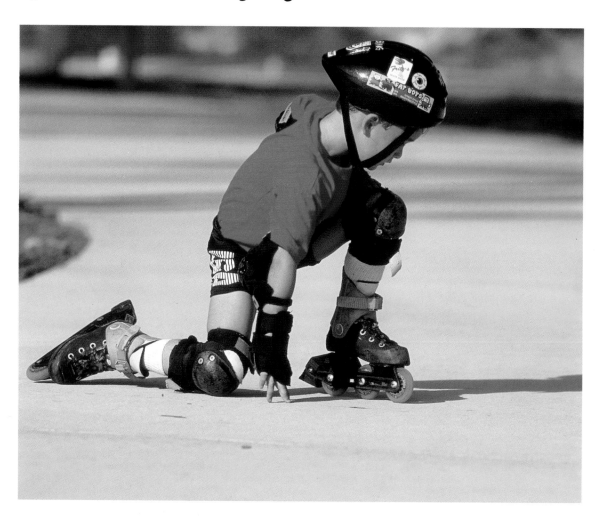

Dancing teaches you how to balance. It also helps make your muscles stronger.

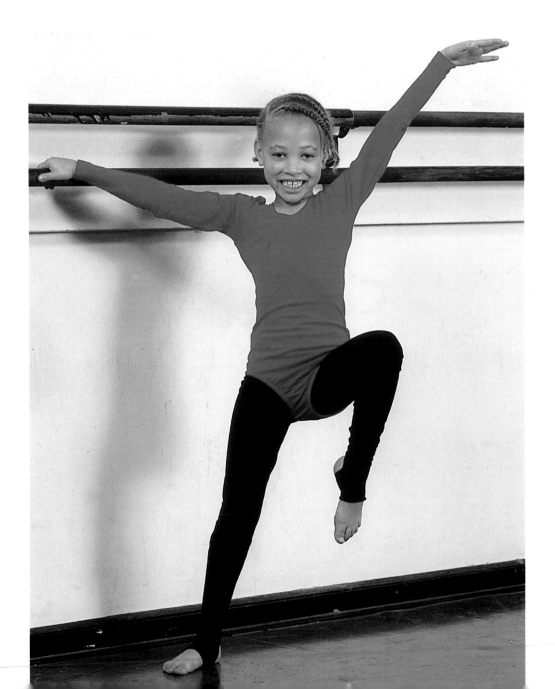

Play Ball

When you throw and catch a ball, you use more than just your **muscles**. Your hands and eyes work together to help you catch the ball.

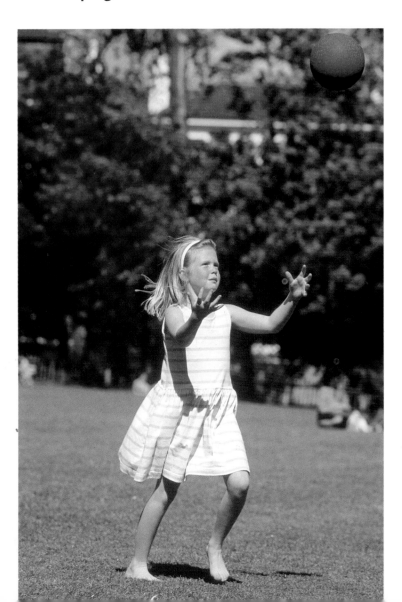

Juggling is even harder! It takes a lot of practice to **coordinate** your eyes and hands like this.

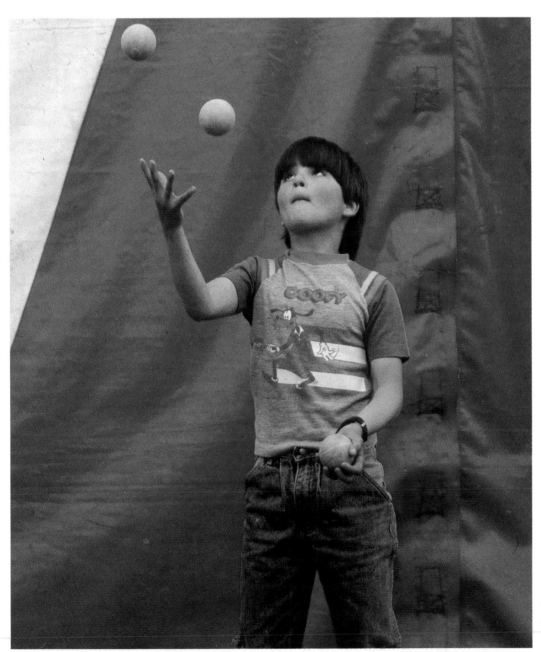

All Together

Cycling uses **muscle** power, balance, and **coordination**. A bicycle ride with your family can be lots of fun.

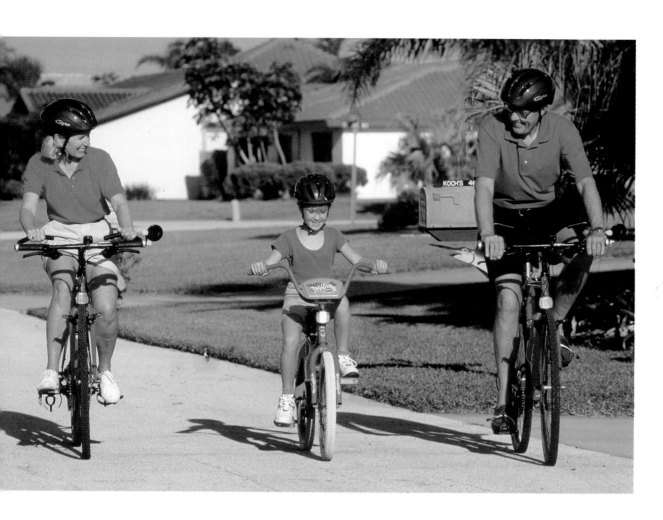

The more you **exercise**, the more fit you get. If you are fit, you can exercise longer without getting tired.

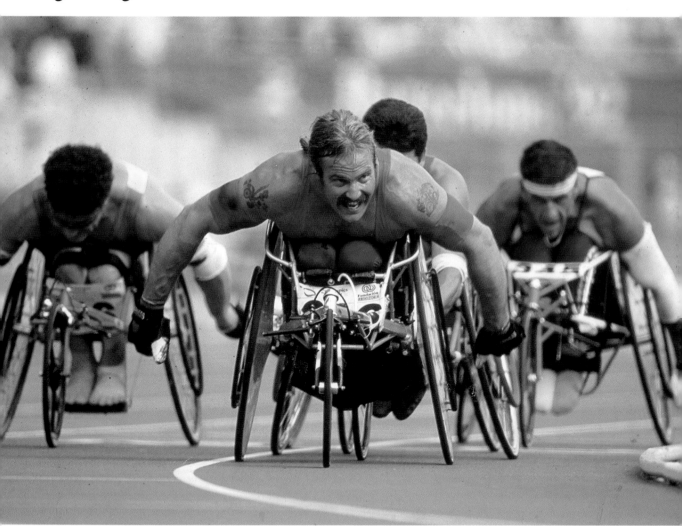

Resting and Playing

To stay fit, you need to **exercise** every day. Walk, take the stairs, or ride your bike whenever you can. Even a little exercise does your body a lot of good.

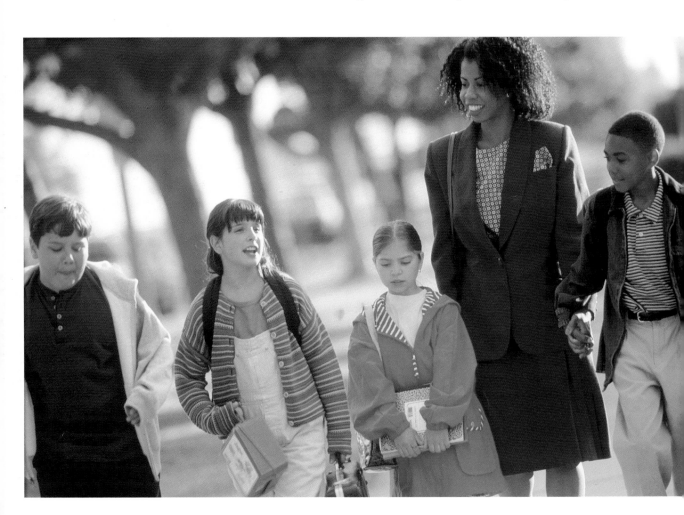

No matter how fit you are, you need to rest sometimes. Sleep well. Your body is getting ready for another busy day!

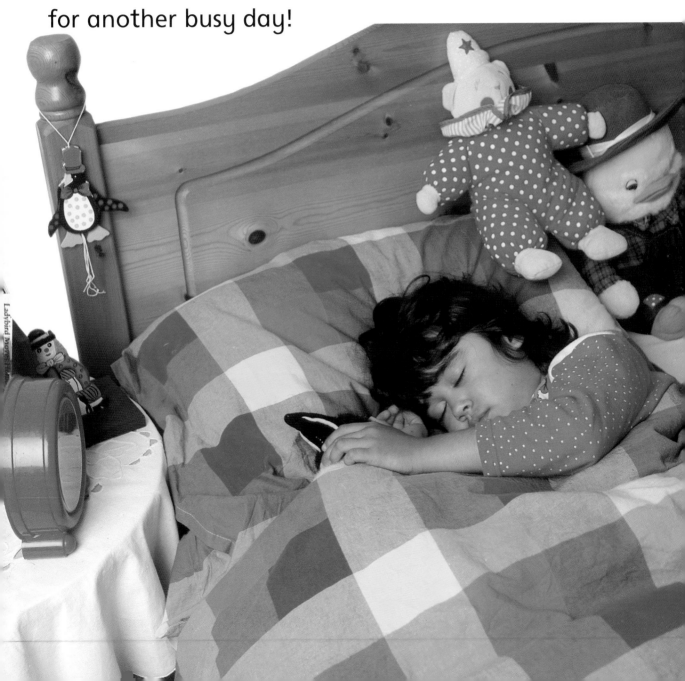

Glossary

activity   something you do while you are moving around

aerobic   making the body better able to use oxygen

blood   red liquid that carries food and oxygen around the body

bone   hard part of the body. Bones are connected to give your body its shape.

coordinate   make different things work together

coordination   when different parts of the body work together to do something

exercise   something you do that uses your muscles and makes your body stronger and more fit

flexible able to bend easily

heart body part that pumps blood around the body

joint place where two bones meet that allows you to bend your arm, leg, or other body parts

lung part of the body used for breathing

muscle part of the body that moves the bones

oxygen gas that makes up part of the air. All living things need oxygen to stay alive.

pyramid shape with a flat bottom and triangle sides that come together in a point at the top.

Index

More Books to Read

Cromwell, Sharon. *Why Can't I Fly?* Des Plaines, Ill.: Rigby Interactive Library, 1998.

McGinty, A. and B. *Staying Healthy: Let's Exercise.* New York: Rosen Publishing Group, 1997.

Powell, Jillian. *Exercise & Your Health.* Austin, Tex.: Raintree Steck-Vaughn, 1998.